Self-Help Toolkit For Anxiety And Stress

Self-Help Toolkit For Anxiety And Stress

A series of simple steps to improve your day and build resiliance against anxiety and stress.

Hayley Bennett

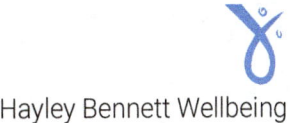

Hayley Bennett Wellbeing

CONTENTS

DEDICATION ix

Disclaimer 1

Introduction 3

Build your resilience to Stress and Anxiety

1 | It can all work out for the best in the end 9

2 | What is Happiness? 13

3 | What are Stress and Anxiety? 23

4 | Let's be grateful! 33

5 | What sort of day will I 'decide' to have today? 41

CONTENTS

6 | What is draining me? 51

7 | The Balance Wheel 61

8 | Reflection, Realisation and Relaxation 71

9 | The tools for your toolkit 79

Working towards the life you want

Introduction 87

10 | Know your vision 89

11 | Know the consequences of not achieving your vision 97

12 | Know your reason for your vision! 101

13 | Know and understand the things that are holding you back. 105

14 | Know your plan. 113

CONTENTS

Notes:

Notes:

Notes:

Bibliography

Acknowledgments

ABOUT THE AUTHOR **133**
WHAT IS LIVE BETTER – FEEL BETTER – WORK BETTER? **135**
WHAT IS SHIFT – CREATION COACHING? **137**
WHAT IS REFLEXOLOGY? **139**

Copyright © 2021 by Hayley Bennett

All rights reserved. No part of this book may be reproduced in any manner whatsoever without written permission except in the case of brief quotations embodied in critical articles and reviews.

First Printing, 2021

I dedicate this book to all the clients I have seen over the years. I have learnt so much from you all.

Disclaimer

The information and recommendations in this book are based on my experience, reading, training undertaken and modalities I am licensed to use. It does not constitute medical advice and is not intended to replace medical advice.

It is important to discuss lifestyle changes with your medical practitioner, especially if you have a pre-existing medical or psychological condition. The application of the information in this book should always be used on the basis of common-sense approach to your own circumstances.

The author disclaims all liability for the use of information in this book.

Introduction

"I'm tired of feeling stressed and unable to find a way out."

"I know I struggle with anxiety but I don't know how to deal with it."

"Everything feels overwhelming and I just can't cope, (no one helps)"

"I know I get a little stressed and anxious, but I'm not depressed so it's OK."

Can you relate, or are you one of those people that feel anxiety, stress and depression is something someone else has, it's something you consider shameful and don't discuss?

Stress and anxiety can creep up on us, we don't have to be in a crisis or a trauma for it to happen, a build-up of things that happen in our lives can become too much if we've not had time to fully recover from them. The next thing we know is we're being negative and not even realising it, something wasn't good enough, something wasn't sorted quick enough, something wasn't to your liking, etc. the spiral has started.

Over the years anxiety and stress have come in and out of my life, they have even taken over sometimes with panic attacks in my younger years and then as I got older, I would get stuck in negative thinking and not see any good in the situation. There have been some low and dark places where I felt like there wasn't a way out. I started to notice that the more I understood about how it was affecting me, the easier it became to deal with, even control. I was learning the signs.

I started to understand more about the brain (medically as well as consciously and unconsciously) to help me with the side effects after having a car accident but it also helped me understand how stress and my mind were causing a lot of my problems.

In this book I have broken down all my knowledge, research and training into simple bite size sections and added some of the tools and techniques I use with my clients to help them control their anxiety and stress. Not all the tools and techniques will be right for you, but that's OK. As you work through the book and exercises, collect the ones that work for you, even if they are ones, you may only use once or twice a year. Collect and create your own Self-Help toolkit, so you can build your resilience and maintain a calm and balanced life.

Resilience
What does resilience mean to you?
Does it mean you can.........

BOUNCE BACK **BE STRONG**

COPE WITH THINGS   **KEEP GOING**

DEAL WITH THINGS   **NOT GIVE UP**

A Look at the *Oxford English Dictionary's* Definition of Resilience:

Resilience is *'The capacity to recover quickly after something unpleasant, such as shock, injury, etc, or the ability of a substance or object to spring back into shape.'*

Read this again.

I don't believe we have to recover quickly; I believe we have to do it in our own time, but we do need to recover, we can't push it away and not deal with it. We need to take steps, small or big to build resilience and recover.

Resilience is not a personality trait; you are not born with it. It is a combination of behaviours, thoughts and action that can be learnt and developed.

Let's take the first step and start building your resilience.

Build your resilience to Stress and Anxiety

Part One

1

It can all work out for the best in the end

We hear it all the time; "It will all work out for the best, in the end" or "You will look back on this and laugh".

At the time you want to tell the other person to go away and leave you alone (and that's the polite version). How can they not see how bad it is, how stressed I am, how anxious I am.

But it can be true; it can be one of the best things that has happened, but how?

I get asked all the time, "Why did I choose to become a Wellbeing practitioner?" Well, my story is one of those that when something bad happened, it turned out to be one of the best things in my life.

When I was 15 years old, I remember flying to Portugal with my family. While we were there, we went to see my uncle and auntie, who were living over there. My auntie had been a healer and doing reflexology for years and my uncle had just learnt to do Reiki and Hypnosis after having cancer. This was all exciting to me and I found it fascinating, but at 15 (back in 1989),

I couldn't really go to the career adviser and ask to be a healer – it wasn't the thing to do; a secretary or working in the bank were the careers they were still pushing. So, I went against the grain. No, I didn't become a healer but I went into design and trained as a Graphic Designer. But just as I was leaving college and had been offered a job at my work placement, I had a car accident.

As much as it was a major accident, myself and my partner at the time, (later to become my husband and the father of my son), were trapped in the burning car, we got out with what appeared to be minor injuries. John, had the horrible memory of the whole experience. Myself, I don't remember any of it as I hit my head and was out cold. John had sat on my lap, kicked the door open and dragged me out. I was X-rayed, stitched up and sent home the next day with broken ribs, sternum, finger and 15 stitches in my head. I could speak, knew my name and the people around me, I was going to be fine or so we thought.

(This is one of those moments when you want to tell the other person to go away!): My uncle from Portugal called and said to me; "The universe obviously has other plans for you"...... Really!!!

The headaches stayed, my balance was off and my memory wasn't great. Every time I tried to get on with my life and go back to work, I would relapse, the headaches got worse, my recall and short-term memory didn't improve and I had started to black out. This went on for quite a few years until I had a really bad relapse after my son was born. They told me I would probably never work again and now I couldn't even look after my son. I felt so useless, what was the point, I just wanted my life to end. But luckily, I was introduced to the Headway charity and I met a great doctor there, who helped me to understand what was going on with my head and gave me the best advice, these few simple words changed my life; *'This illness will control your life, unless you learn to control it!'*

I couldn't let this illness rule my life, I needed to take control and learn how to work with it, not against it.

I went back to what I had found fascinating on that trip to Portugal; I turned to alternative treatments and started to understand my body and mind. Over time I realised one of the big problems I had was my mindset. I wanted to be the 'Hayley' I was before the accident, so every time I pushed myself to become that person, I pushed myself too far and then crashed. I was on a roller coaster; I needed to stop the ride and find out where my limits were. I needed to be the new 'Hayley', the one I was now after the accident and stay more stable.

I'm not saying this was easy or that it happened overnight. It took me a long time but slowly I figured it out. I learnt about a balanced life, I learnt what foods worked for me, about how exercise helped me mentally and physically and I learnt to listen to my body and to be kind to myself.

'Know when to stop, don't follow the crowd, do what is right for you!'

This was a hard thing to do. I was changing, I was going in a different direction and I couldn't keep up with the pace. The other people in my life were still on the same path I had been on with them before the accident. This was a point in my life when I couldn't see how this accident (the bad thing) could be the best thing that had happened to me. I was finding what was best for me, but losing things around me.

As I became more balanced in my life, the better I felt and slowly over the years I took on a little more. In 2002 I trained as a reflexologist and I have never looked back. My life and my job worked hand in hand. The more I trained, the more I understood my life and illness, and the more I understood the more I could put it into my life and the more I could help others because I was living it. I was living proof!

Sharing my knowledge and tools, helping people on their life journey is a job I love and I couldn't do it as well as I do if it wasn't for the accident.

Maybe this was what my uncle meant with 'The universe has other plans for you'

We all have things we have to deal with in life and some of us hide them away but if we look at things differently, we will be able to see the good that can come from them. Don't see limitations as negative things, see them as an alternative, maybe a better way, even if they are different.

I might have limitations and I have to stick to a few rules to have a functioning life. But I'm upright and I'm living my life to the full.

2

What is Happiness?

What is happiness?

It might seem like an odd question, but is it?

Do you know how to define happiness?

Do you think happiness is the same thing to you as it is to others?

Does happiness even make a difference in your life?

In fact, happiness does have a pretty important role in our lives, and it can have a huge impact on the way we live. Although researchers have yet to pin down the definition or an agreed-upon framework for happiness, there's a lot we have learned in the last few decades.

In 2013 I attended the *'Coaching Happiness'* course with Robert Holden. Robert Holden is a British psychologist, author, and broadcaster, who works in the field of positive psychology and well-being and is considered "Britain's foremost expert on happiness". He is the founder of the "Happiness Project", which runs an eight-week course annually, called "Happiness Now" and the author of 10 best-selling books such as, Happiness NOW! Be Happy, Success Intelligence and Shift Happens! The minute I heard his talk from the Hay House convention on a podcast, I knew I needed to train with him. It was funny, a friend had been to the convention in the USA and had bought the download of all the talks that had happed at the event, she had been raving about the convention for days, so I borrowed the download and started to listen to the different talks. I remember, I was painting my treatment room and thought it was a great way to keep me entertained, so, I plugged in my headphones to listen away, but every talk I listen to was either something I already knew about, not interested in or I couldn't stand their voice. I was living in Bermuda and I was getting use to the American accent as we heard it on the TV and a lot of Americans holidayed in Bermuda, but some of the accents were too hard on my hearing and I couldn't concentrate. I flicked through the talks, listened to a bit, then moved on until I heard an English accent, this I could listen to. It's funny how you start to crave little things from home when you live away.

It wasn't just his accent, it was what he was saying, it was resonating with me. Things I had learnt along my journey, both in my personal life and in my career, were being talked about by a psychologist. He was putting research and facts together with how I thought and how I was trying to teach my clients. I listened and re-listened to his talk. I bought his books, followed his website and then I saw his training in San Diego and never looked back. I had made a shift in my career.

Let's take a look at the definition of happiness so we're all on the same page. *Oxford English Dictionary*'s definition of *"happiness"* is a simple one:

"*The state of being happy.*"

Not exactly what we were looking for, was it? Perhaps we need to dive a little deeper. *Oxford English Dictionary*'s definition of *"happy"* is a little more helpful:

"*Feeling or showing pleasure or contentment.*"

So, happiness is the state of feeling or showing pleasure or contentment. From this definition, we can glean a few important points about happiness:

1. Happiness is a state, not a trait; in other words, it isn't a long-lasting, permanent feature or personality trait, but a more fleeting, changeable state.
2. Happiness is equated with feeling pleasure or contentment, meaning that happiness is not to be confused with joy, ecstasy, bliss, or other more intense feelings.
3. Happiness can be either feeling or showing, meaning that happiness is not necessarily an internal or external experience, but can be both.

Is it difficult to define scientifically?

With so many takes on happiness, it's no wonder that happiness is a little difficult to define scientifically; there is certainly disagreement about what, exactly, happiness is. Although they generally all agree on what happiness feels like - being satisfied with life, in a good mood, feeling positive emotions, feeling enjoyment, etc. -researchers have found it difficult to agree on the scope of happiness.

The *OED*'s definition combined with that of positive psychologists:
"Happiness is a state characterized by contentment and general satisfaction with one's current situation."

With all this in mind, why has society in recent years gathered pace and our stress levels have gone through the roof? We have become increasingly obsessed with money, job titles, appearances and an endless accumulation of stuff, which we need NOW! And if it's not there now, we are disappointed or frustrated. There is a growing sense of discontent as we push ourselves harder and juggle more. We are overworked, overstretched and overwhelmed, but not stopping to see why.

We just believe this is normal. We live in a culture of more:

MORE FREEDOM   **MORE CHOICE**

MORE CONVENIENCE   **MORE POTENTIAL**

MORE OPPORTUNITIES   **MORE MONEY**

MORE INCOME   **MORE STORAGE**

MORE EXPECTATIONS

In today's world we are being told we need more, but the more we get the more we need. We buy new clothes when we don't need them, we need a better car to look like we're doing well, we need that bigger house, that new kitchen, that new sofa when there isn't anything wrong with the other one. This merry-go-round goes from a calm, joyful ride to a never-ending treadmill. We start off enjoying the excitement of the new 'more' but then it becomes something we are trying to keep up with because we feel it makes you happy and we are worried if you ever stop everything will come tumbling down.

Happiness - Research has shown that people believe that their happiness depends on something else, they say it will come when:

- I have more money
- I have more success
- I have a new car
- I have a bigger house
- I have a new hair style and look like someone famous or just everyone else
- I have that new top, new dress, new coat

We have more but are we happier?
Or are we just semi happy?

Semi Happy

The *Urban Dictionary* Definition of Semi happy.
"*A not so happy emotion that makes you have anxiety and stress*".
So, it is kind of messing with people.

When we are semi happy, we do something to distract ourselves from facing the fact that we are not fully happy. We '*feel*', we consciously convince ourselves, that if we have this or do this thing now it will make us happy; we have learnt to use short term fixes to mask our unhappiness
We.........

Buy something   Eat Something   Work some more

Drink some more   Push ourselves more

Earn some more money   Buy Something

Eat something......

We are creating lives we feel we regularly want to escape from with a Large Gin and Tonic and a Cigarette or a Bubble

Bath and Chocolate, instead of creating a life we want to live everyday.

Static Happiness and Semi Happy

Ever since happiness researchers have measured happiness and well-being levels they have noticed an interesting phenomenon: in spite of the fact that we have more of everything we say we want; we are not any happier. Research has shown that over 60 years we have static happiness. Studies in the US asked a hundred people to mark out of ten how happy they are. Ten being very happy. This shows static happiness.

US
1950's - 7.5 out of 10 people were happy
2010's - 7.4 out of 10 people were happy

In the UK they asked a hundred people how happy they are. This shows we are also now only semi happy.

UK
1957 - 52% of people were very happy
2017 - 37% of people were very happy

This is interesting the percentage of people that are happy has dropped but we live in a time where we all have more!

Average ratings of happiness in the UK fell by 1.1% in the year ending March 2020, this was before Covid-19 had started. England was the only country of the UK to experience a significant reduction in average life satisfaction ratings (0.6%) between the first quarter (Jan to Mar) of 2019 and the first quarter of 2020.

Latest data in relation to Mental Health and Covid -19. All data has been extracted from: The office of National Statistics, all adults Great Britain. - 13th-17th January 2021.

Personal well-being scores remain at some of the lowest levels ever since this year's survey began back in March 2020 and the feeling of happiness is dropping each week.

Was this because people were unable to have quick, short-term fixes? no going out getting drunk, no going to the shops to distract themselves and no eating out with friends. They were all at home, with time and space to face the underlying problems of their unhappiness.

Jaggi Vasudev, known publicly as **Sadhguru**, is an Indian yogi and author, who says:

> *Those who are happy, know how to be happy*

But being happy isn't the problem, we've all been happy. The problem is maintaining it, we struggle to maintain happiness.

If you look back on the last 24 hours, how many times have you been happy, how many moments of joy have you had?

Count on your fingers, 1-2-5?

For some people it's 0, there is nothing to be happy about.

When you were a child, a 5-year-old, how many moments of joy did you have in 24 hours? Lots of them. Someone had to make you unhappy.

Now someone has to make you happy!

Sadhguru, goes on to say the reverse has happened, we have lost our happiness. If we were so happy at 5-years old, we should be ecstatic by the time we become 30, but we're not. We believe our personal journey is the be-all and end-all of life itself, our personal achievements, ownership and our looks define the universe.

He says we've lost all connection to who we are and the real fundamental reason for living and being happy.

As someone who has spent the best part of two decades helping people manage their health and their lives, so they can live better and feel better. Over the years I have seen how so many of us are making ourselves ill with over-commitment, constant comparison, judgement and negative self-talk. We are sleepwalking through our days, spending too much time cooped up in our boxes dulling our senses, paying attention to celebrities, advertising and social media rather than exploring our own lives and feelings and seeing the rich potential they have.

> *We give away freely that most precious of resources – our attention, and in doing so, we cheat ourselves out of the gifts that are already here. – Beth Kempton.*

But on a positive note, for some time now, I have been hearing people say they want something different. There's a growth of understanding and a yearning for a simpler, more meaningful life. Now, after 2020 and COVID-19 people are wanting this more. They are looking for a life infused with beauty, a connection to nature, an energy of everyday wellbeing, built around what matters most to them. The more people come to me exhausted, stuck, unwell and unhappy, the more I felt I needed to share my knowledge and tools that have helped me to live a more authentic and inspired life.

In this book we will work together to build your resilience to life's circumstances through behaviour, thoughts and actions, so you can be happy and work towards a life you want.

3

What are Stress and Anxiety?

Most people experience stress and anxiety from time to time.

Stress is any demand placed on your brain or physical body. People can report feeling stressed when multiple competing demands are placed on them. The feeling of being stressed can be triggered by an event that makes you feel frustrated or nervous.

Stress is wanting the present moment to be something it's not.

Anxiety is a feeling of fear, worry, or unease. It can be a reaction to stress, or it can occur in people who are unable to identify significant stressors in their life.

Anxiety is creating a narrative in the mind of what *might* happen and then staying focused on it. By staying focused on the story in our head, our emotions kick in (example; Fear) and then reinforces the narrative.

Anxiety is a general term for several disorders that cause nervousness, fear, apprehension, and worrying. These disorders affect how we feel and behave and can cause physical symptoms. Mild anxiety is vague and unsettling, while severe anxiety can seriously affect day-to-day living.

Anxiety disorders affect over 8 million people in the UK. That means 1 in 6 adults suffer with it. It is the most common group of mental illnesses in the country. However, only 36.9 percent of people with the condition receive treatment.

Stress and anxiety are not always bad. In the short-term, they can help you overcome a challenge or dangerous situation. Examples of everyday stress and anxiety include worrying about finding a job, feeling nervous before a big test, or being embarrassed in certain social situations. If we did not experience some stress or anxiety, we might not be motivated to do things that we need to do (for instance, studying for that big test!).

So, if this is true, *stress and anxiety isn't always bad!* Why is it taking over so many peoples live and how does it become bad for us? This is where I need to go into more detail, break it all down to explain what it does to us, our bodies and our minds. By reading the next section you will be able to understand how long-term stress and anxiety takes over and you will see how it triggers us, so we can learn to manage it.

What is Fight or Flight and how does it have anything to do with stress and anxiety?

Without your fight or flight system, you'd probably do nothing. You wouldn't be able to fear the danger and the mind and the body wouldn't know that you needed to run away from that danger. Even if you did, you'd have nothing helping you. It would be like getting into a fight but being unable to use much strength or respond very quickly.

That's why you have a fight or flight response. That response is a flood of changes to your hormones and neurotransmitters, it prepares your body to immediately run away or fight. It's designed to cover all of the bases: improving blood flow to the areas that need it, keeping your body cool, providing you with more energy, helping you see and respond more quickly, improving your mindset, etc.

Thanks to the fight or flight system, you'd immediately know to feel fear when you see the danger, you'd have the energy to run away, and you wouldn't hurt your body in the process. The fight or flight system is actually one of the most important tools that your body has, even though these days most people rarely face too much danger.

But what we do face in the world today is stress and this kicks off the fight and flight system. The only difference is that so many don't come down from the fight or flight high. When fight or flight happens the cortisol level in the blood is pumped around the body and to the brain. We are then meant to come down from the cortisol high after the act is over.

We see danger, the cortisol level kicks in, we fight or fly and then the body calms down.

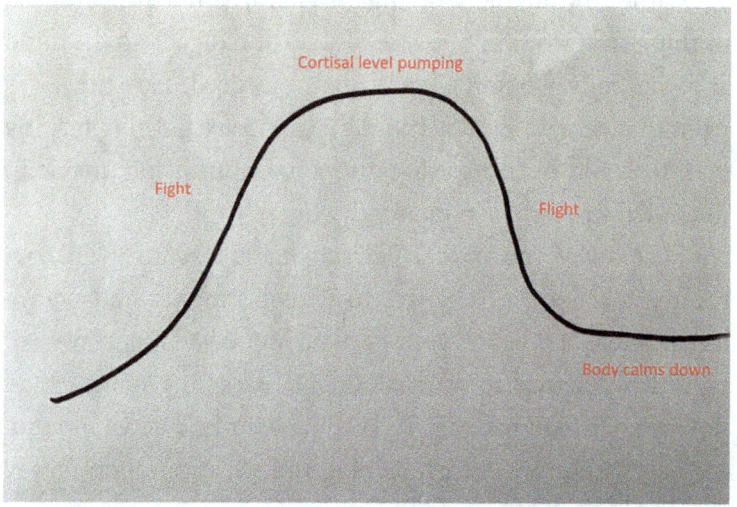

But with long term stress, we are not getting the chance to calm down, we are on the go, the 'more' must still happen.

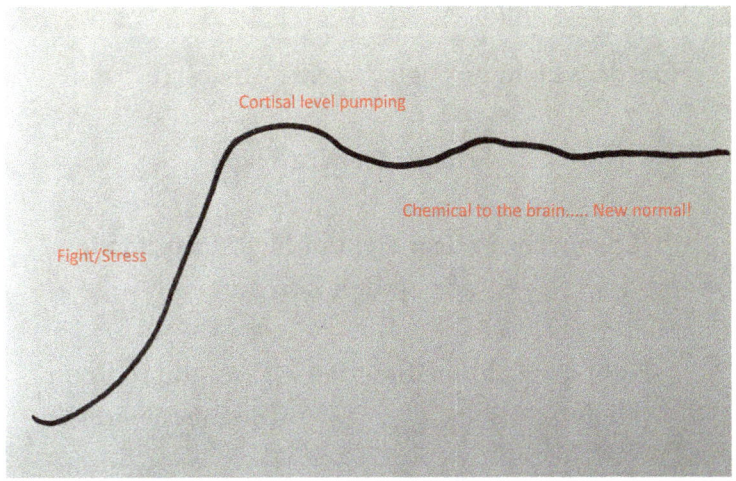

When this keeps happening the body sends a chemical to the brain telling the brain this is normal. We start to think it is normal but while all this is happening the rest of the body is working overtime, e.g., adrenal glands, spleen and kidneys, these organs play a part to keeping our immune system strong.

The immune system is a complex network of cells and proteins that defends the body against infection. The body can't run like this for long periods without getting depleted, your fight or flight system affects your glucose levels and uses adrenaline to provide your body with a flood of energy, which causes you to shake. Also issues in the digestive system and bladder areas as the fight or flight response slows digestion and weakens your bladder because these systems are not prioritised in this response. One reason so many people are becoming ill and run down is that their immune systems are suppressed by long term stress.

How does Fight or Flight become Anxiety?

Stress = Fight or Flight

Long term stress = Fight or Flight malfunction (High Cortisol)

Fight or Flight malfunction = Chemical to Brain
(High Cortisol)   (Becomes Normal)

Long term Chemical to Brain = Cloudy Brain
(Normal)   (Toxic)

So, if the body is suffering from anxiety or stress for a long period the brain gets cloudy, as you can see hormones and toxins are sent to the brain, this is toxic and the brain is unable to think or see clearly. You are unable to think straight or make the right decision and you feel overwhelmed, but you don't realise you are unable to think straight because your brain is cloudy. The cortisol your body releases, acts as a shield and cuts off access to the frontal lobe, the rational thinking part of the brain. Now this is when the anxiety will kick in and the cycle begins.

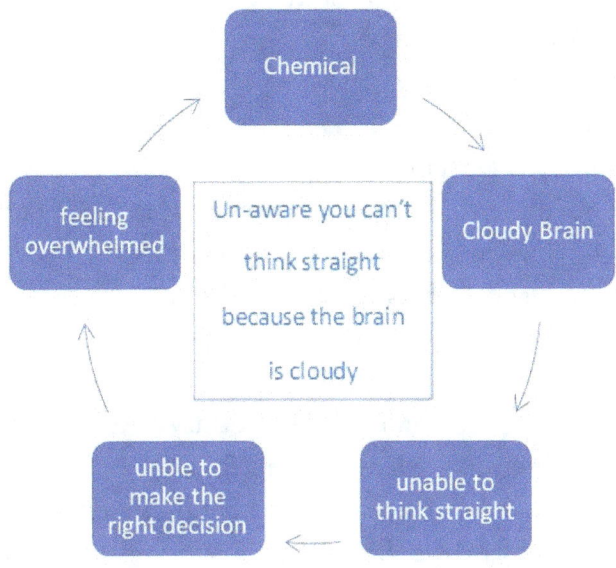

All these reactions are why we get symptoms from being stressed or suffering with anxiety.

Symptoms

There are several different types of anxiety and stress, each with a distinct set of symptoms. However, common symptoms can include:

- Sweating
- Dizziness
- Trembling

- Increased or irregular heartbeat
- Back pain
- Restlessness and fatigue
- Muscle tension
- Being easily startled
- Recurring and ongoing feelings of worry, with or without known stressors
- Avoidance of certain situations that may cause worry, often affecting quality of life.

Long term stress and anxiety you may have some of the above symptoms as well as a more nagging sense of fear. You may experience being irritable, have trouble sleeping, develop headaches, or have trouble getting on with work and planning for the future. Your sex life maybe affected and might lose self-confidence.

Positive psychologists say that stress, anxiety and worry are likely to be felt by those whose lives are high in meaningfulness and low in happiness; this indicates that you shouldn't get too down about experiencing negative emotions if you have a strong sense of meaning – a little negative emotion can actually be a good thing.

If we start to understand what the anxiety and low moods do to us, we can start to work with *it*, instead of *it* working against us. There are 4 ways it can affect us; *Thoughts, Emotion, Physical symptoms and Behaviours*. The *Thoughts* are the unrealistic and negative thinking, The *Emotions* are the feelings we feel, The *Physical symptoms* are how it comes out in the body and The *Behaviours* are how we react to the situation.

Take a look at the lists below for some common symptoms of anxiety and low mood.

Under each section there are different symptoms. Tick which ones you experience, so you can see how it affects you.

How does anxiety affect you?

Thoughts	Emotion
"Something awful is going to happen"	Anxious
"I will not be able to cope"	Scared
"What if I don't do it right"	Nervous
"What will people think of me"	Irritable
"I need to escape"	Depressed

Physical Symptoms	Behaviours
Faster heart beat	Avoiding situations
Physical tension	Increased smoking or drinking
Dizziness	Arguing
Hot and sweaty	Talking or doing things faster
Tunnel vision	Under or over eating

How does low mood affect you?

Thoughts	Emotions
"I'm a failure"	Depressed
"People think I'm stupid"	Sad
"Nobody Likes me"	Lethargic
"I might as well not be here"	Irritable
"There's no point, I won't enjoy it"	Suicidal

Physical Symptoms	Behaviours
Difficulties sleeping	Social withdrawal
Poor appetite or over eating	Increased smoking or drinking
Tearful	Decrease in activities
Loss of sex drive	Sleeping during the day

However, if stress and anxiety begin interfering with your daily life, it may indicate a more serious issue. If you are avoiding situations due to fears, constantly worrying, or experiencing severe anxiety about a traumatic event weeks after it happened, it may be time to seek help.

When we actively practice anxiety and stress management techniques to stay calm, we can access the rational thinking part of the brain and start to create a clearer and more positive outlook.

In the next chapter we start to build your toolkit to help manage your stress and anxiety.

4

Let's be grateful!

We have all heard that we need to be grateful for the little things around us, it is a word we hear people using a lot nowadays. But as a child I only ever heard it being mentioned when I heard people praying on the TV around the dinner table; *'I'm thankful for the food that is on the table'*. Being thankful to me meant they were grateful. I'm not saying my parents weren't grateful, they were. I just didn't hear the *'word – grateful'* being used like we do now.

Being grateful can be easier on days when life is going well, it is easier to stop and see the beautiful flowers as you walk along, to notice the person who has held the door open for you, to notice the work colleague that had made you a coffee as they saw you working hard. But when your day or week isn't going so well it can be harder to pick up on these things. We feel overwhelmed, like everything is going wrong and we can't see the good or positive in anything.

If we start being grateful on the good days it will become a habit and then it becomes easier on the harder days. Even in the depth of sadness we can find something to be grateful for, we might not want to but it is there.

For example: We could be grieving over a loss but still see we have support around us and be grateful for those people.

This doesn't make the grieving or loss go away but it does stop us feeling alone and that feeling helps us see a way forward.

To be grateful we first need to understand what it means.

Dictionary.com definition of *Grateful* is a warmly or deeply appreciative of kindness or benefits received; *thankful:* I am *grateful* to you for your help; expressing *gratitude*: a *grateful* letter; pleasing to the mind or senses; agreeable or welcome; refreshing: a *grateful* breeze.

Gratitude is a warm feeling of thankfulness towards the world, or towards specific individuals. The person who feels *gratitude* is *thankful* for what they have, and does not constantly seek more.

Research shows that people who are grateful tend to show a higher level of well-being and happiness; in other words, they feel better about themselves and their lives. In return this improves their mental health and can even help them sleep better

Expressing gratitude to others, those who have given us something, whether that is out of the goodness of their heart or in the line of duty, helps them to feel good and improves their self-esteem.

Gratitude has been shown to improve social ties and promotes more social behaviour. It makes other people want to show more gratitude too, a phenomenon known as 'Upstream reciprocity'. Grateful people tend to want to repay a favour, and not just to the person who did them the favour but to other people as well. In Bermuda, a country I lived in for 10 years, they teach their children to give back to the community. They start at the age of 12 doing community service through the school. As they get older the number of hours increase. By the time they are leaving at 18 they will have done 150 hours of community service per year for the previous 2 years. This teaches them gratitude for what they have and that if they help others, it can have a huge effect on those people. In some Eastern religions, including Hinduism and Buddhism this is known as Karma, a Sanskrit word that roughly translates to *"Action"*. Karma generally indicates the cycle of cause and effect, what goes out, must come back, good or bad.

Being grateful for the things around us, the things we already have, will help us stay focused on the positive, not the negative. i.e., the things that could go wrong, the things we don't have, etc. By staying focused on the positive, the good, the nice things, the happy things, we calm the mind and the action part of the brain. In return we are in a better position to cope with things that are thrown at us and the things that change in our lives. We start to train the brain to see the good in things and the good in change. It also helps us to be happy with what we have, even when things aren't so good. It slows the process of needing more to be happy.

NOW IS THE NEW BEGINNING

> **THE HAPPIEST PEOPLE DON'T HAVE THE BEST OF EVERYTHING.**
> **THEY JUST MAKE THE BEST OF EVERYTHING.**

Each day for the next 5 days I invite you to write down 5 things that you are grateful for. They can be big or small e.g. my Health, my family, the sweet my child shared with me, my neighbour stopping to say 'Hi' this morning, seeing the butterfly on my walk. If you have more than 5 then keep writing but if you're struggling to think of things, start to look at the little stuff. This will help you to see that there are lots of great things happening to you each day. It also helps pull you out of the drama and stress that you can get caught up in. It makes you take a step back, gives you time to breathe and refocus.

Day 1 - Toolkit

Start your day with 5 things you are grateful for:

1

2

3

4

5

About my Day

Looking back at your day can be very helpful, it can help you see what went well and what didn't. I'm not asking you to criticise and beat yourself up when the day didn't go well or you didn't handle something well. It's more about seeing the things that work for you and remembering them so you can use them another time. When you notice the things that trigger you, they can be an opportunity for learning. When things go wrong, you can learn and find a new way of handling the situation.

Ask yourself these questions:

- What is triggering me?
- Why is it triggering me?
- What can I do to change the outcome?
- Do I need to remove myself from the situation so it doesn't happen again?

Complete the questions below at the **END** of your day so you can start to break down your day and find the things you need and don't need and the tools that work for you.

Today was a good/bad day for me because....

What did I learn from my day?

What can I change for tomorrow?

What 3 things am I grateful for from my day.

1

2

3

Taking time out from your day is a great way to relax and let go of your stresses, even a few minutes can make a big difference.

Sit and Breathe

- Begin by sitting comfortably and close your eyes.
- Make sure you sit upright and drop your shoulder blades down your back and your shoulders away from your ears.

- Feel the chest open up.
- **Take a few deep breaths** – take a deep breath in and as you let it all out, make a noise. Loud and long, allow all your tension, worries, fears and negativity out with the breath.
- Repeat this a few times and feel the tension release out of your body and mind.

Meditation - The Bubble

This meditation can be used when you feel you need some protection and strength to deal with your day or a situation

- Begin by sitting comfortably and close your eyes.
- Take a few deep breaths
- Imagine a **Golden bubble** coming around you, this is your safe place.
- Now imagine a **light positive** colour coming into your bubble.
- Breathe in the light positive colour and allow this to fill your body.
- This bubble is your **safe place**, it will give you strength and control over how you feel.

5

What sort of day will I 'decide' to have today?

This was a big lesson for me. I was one of those people that allowed what happened in my day to control how I felt. If I'd had a bad day with my son, or I had an argument with my partner, I would feel my life was a mess; I was no good and then I'd feel unhappy.

We can also turn it around and blame others, the economy, our partners or kids, the calories, the government, work or even God. If you are ever tempted to blame anyone for your lack of happiness you would do well to look in the mirror first.

Being accountable for your happiness, or lack of it, is an important step in attracting more happiness.

Here are a few of the main ways we limit our happiness:

Self-Criticism   **Self-Neglect**

Self-Deception   **Self-Alienation**

Self-Doubt   Self-Exhaustion

Self-Control

All of these come from Negative - Automatic - Thoughts or NATs

NATs are thoughts that seem to just pop into our head without warning, they often trigger negative feelings and drive our unhealthy behaviours in an unhelpful direction.

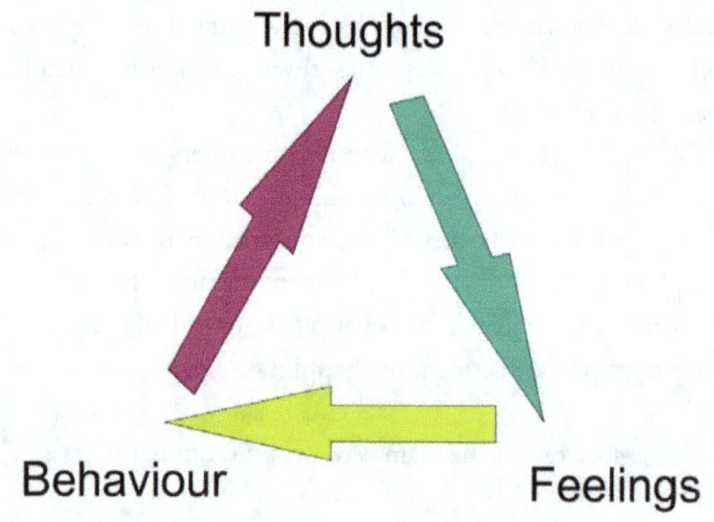

The Big Four Types of Negative Thinking

- **All-or-Nothing Thinking:** "I have to do things perfectly, and anything less is a failure."
- **Focusing on the Negatives:** "Nothing goes my way. It feels like one disappointment after another." A variation of this is being overly judgmental: "The world is falling apart. I don't like what I see around me."
- **Negative Self-Labelling:** "I'm a failure. If people knew the real me, they wouldn't like me. I am flawed."
- **Catastrophizing:** "If something is going to happen, it'll probably be the worst-case scenario."

Other Common Types of Negative Thinking

- **Excessive Need for Approval:** "I can only be happy if people like me. If someone is upset, it's probably my fault."
- **Mind Reading:** "I can tell people don't like me because of the way they behave."
- **'Should' Statements:** "People should be fair, and when they are not, they should be punished."
- **Disqualifying the Present:** "I'll relax later. But first I have to rush to finish this."
- **Dwelling on the Past:** "If I dwell on why, I'm unhappy and what went wrong, maybe I'll feel better."
- **Pessimism:** "Life is a struggle. I don't think we are meant to be happy. I don't trust people who are happy. If some-

thing good happens in my life, I usually have to pay for it with something bad."

The more we start to understand ourselves and our thoughts, feelings and behaviours the easier it becomes to change them. The better we know ourselves, the better we can survive and build resilience. In chapter 12 and in the bonus section, *working toward your goals and dreams*, we work on how to change your negative thoughts to positive and realistic thoughts.

Thoughts and beliefs can be both positive and negative. A *positive* thought or belief will empower you, whereas a *negative* thought will disempower you. This expresses itself through our internal chatter (what we say to ourselves, our inner voice) and our external chatter (what we express outwardly about ourselves and how we speak to others).

Your brain chemistry changes when you're in a negative state, as we know from chapter 2. Negative thinking traps you and shuts down the brain. Positive empowered thinking floods the brain with serotonin and helps you be more creative, which helps you to find a clear solution to your situation. By holding onto negative thoughts and beliefs you create pain and fear.

Anger comes from pain and fear!

We don't make life easier by not dealing with our fears. We're reliving the pain over and over by pushing it aside. By doing this we can consciously and unconsciously offload our pain on to others. If we don't offload to others, we hold it inside and beat ourselves up. Either way it's an unhealthy behaviour.

> *When we are blinded by anger, we make choices we later regret. We are the ones that get burnt!*

No matter how hurt or angry we are, we don't need to retaliate or have the last word. It is so easy these days to just fire back words of anger in a text or email to someone that has upset us. But are we reacting with a clear head? Do we need to react at all?

Having the last word or being right can obliterate even the good memories.

When someone has sent a text/email or even said something hurtful to you;

1. Stay calm and collected,
2. Breathe for 30 seconds,
3. Remember it is their anger, not yours.

When we fight back and demand "what is your problem" we're spending more time with that unhappy person.

Leaving the room before the bridge is burned is a sign of maturity!

Or we can be the ones lashing the anger out, off-loading your pain on to others. It's easier to offload pain than it is to feel pain – Are *you* hurting others?

Day 2 – Toolkit

Start you day with 5 things you are grateful for:

1

2

3

4

5

Complete the questions below at the **BEGINNING** of your day. By setting an intention on how you want your day to be or what you want to achieve, you focus your energy on it. If you also look at the things you need to help you achieve it and the things that usually stop you, you can find solutions.

This can be as simple as; I decide to be happy, calm, helpful or it can be more detailed; I decide to join in more or do some exercises. Write whatever works for you.

What sort of day will I have today?

What 3 things can you do to help you achieve the sort of day you want.

1

2

3

Do you need anyone else's help to achieve the sort of day you want? If so who?

What negative thoughts do you have that will stop you achieving the sort of day you want?

About my Day

Complete the questions below at the **END** of your day.

Today was a good/bad day for me because....

What did I learn from my day?

What can I change for tomorrow?

What 3 things am I grateful for from my day?

1

2

3

HAYLEY BENNETT

6

What is draining me?

When we feel overwhelmed and tired of life, it is usually because we have too much going on and a pile of stuff we've not dealt with or had time to do. All these things we've put aside can all pile up and can start to drain us mentally, emotionally and physically

I know if I have lots on my to do list, plus family stuff, I can sometimes struggle to sleep, I lay awake, writing lists in my head or I wake up in the night thinking about what I have to do. Having a lack of sleep and a head full of stuff to think about, my brain starts to feel overloaded but when I start to break down what is draining me, that feeling will lift.

" *'Worry gives a small things Big Shadows.'* "

Day 3 – Toolkit

Start your day with 5 things you are grateful for:

1

2

3

4

5

Below is a list of things that could be draining you. Read through the list and tick off anything that is relevant to you.

Relationships

- There are people in my life who continuously drain my energy

- I have unreturned phone calls, e-mails or letters that need to be handled
- I have an unresolved conflict with a family member
- I lack quality friendships in my life
- I feel a void in my life created by the lack of a romantic partner
- There is someone I need to forgive
- There is a relationship I need to end
- There is a phone call I dread making, and it causes me stress & anxiety
- I'm currently involved in a relationship that compromises my values
- I miss being a part of a loving and supportive community

Environment

- My car needs cleaning and/or repair
- My wardrobe needs updating and/or alterations
- I'd like to live in a different geographic location
- I have appliances that need repair or upgrading
- My home is not decorated in a way that nurtures me
- My cupboards are cluttered and need to be cleaned
- Repairs need to be done around my home
- My home is cluttered and disorganised
- I miss having more beauty reflected in my environment
- I watch too much television

Body, Mind & Spirit

- I eat food that's not good for me
- Something about my physical appearance bothers me
- It's been too long since I've been to the dentist
- I do not get the sleep I need to feel fully rested
- I'd like to exercise regularly but never seem to find the time
- I have a health concern for which I've avoided getting help
- I have emotional needs that consistently go unmet
- There are books that I'd love to read but never seem to find the time for
- I lack personal interest that are intellectually stimulating
- I lack a spiritual or religious practice in my life

Work

- I no longer enjoy my job and have a hard time showing up each day
- My work is stressful and leaves me exhausted at the end of the day
- My office is disorganised, my desk is a mess, and I have trouble finding what I need
- I'm avoiding a confrontation or conflict at work
- I tolerate bad behaviour from a boss or colleague

- I am not computer literate, and it gets in the way of my productivity
- I lack the proper office equipment that I need to do my job well
- My work does not allow me to express my creativity
- I know I need to delegate specific tasks but I am unable to let go of control
- I feel overwhelmed with the amount of information that enters my life in the form of mail, books, magazines and e-mail.

Money

- I have tax returns that are not filed or taxes that are not paid
- I pay my bills late
- I spend more than I earn
- I don't have a plan for my financial future
- My credit rating is not what I'd like it to be
- I do not have a regular savings plan
- I do not have adequate insurance coverage
- My mortgage rate is too high and I need to re-finance
- I have debt that needs to be paid off
- My will is not up to date

From 'Take Time for Your Life' by Cheryl Richardson

Some of these things we can change, we can stop and find the time to pay the late bill but there are others that need a little more work and support to achieve them.

This is the point of this exercise, to stop and see where we need help. Asking for help can be one of the hardest things we can do. We all need support in variety shapes and sizes from friends, family, teachers, professionals and strangers.

We need to let go of our ego (only 'I' can do this) or let go of the thought that only one person can help us. We need to start building a network of people and things around to help us get through our day, week, month and year.

Sit and Breathe

I learnt this breathing technique in yoga years ago and it has been pulled out of my toolkit many times.

Alternate Nostril Breathing also referred to as "Channel-clearing Breath," Alternate nostril breathing is a commonly-used breathing technique, or Pranayama. It encourages deep relaxation because it is believed to balance the left and right sides of the brain while calming the nervous system. It relieves anxiety and quiets an unsettled mind.

- Take a few deep breaths
- Allow your left hand to lie face down on your left thigh. Extend your fingers on your right hand like you are waving at someone.

- Bend your peace fingers—pointer and middle finger—so they curl into your palm.
- Rest your right ring finger and thumb on either side of your nostrils, lightly touching them but not constricting.
- Take a big breath in and a big breath out, then close off the right nostril with your thumb and inhale through the left nostril fully for a count of four.
- At the top of that breath, close off the left nostril with your ring finger, hold and retain the breath for a count of four.
- Release the right nostril and exhale for a count of four.
- Inhale deeply for a count of four through the right nostril, close it off, hold and retain the breath for a count of four.
- Release the left nostril as you exhale completely through it for a count of four. Proceed to inhale deeply through the left, repeating the cycle. The count of breath can be as long as you like, keeping the inhales, retention, and exhales even. Do this as many rounds as you like, being sure to exhale through the left nostril to complete your last cycle.

About my Day

Complete the questions below at the **END** of your day.

Today was a good/bad day for me because....

What did I learn from my day?

What can I change for tomorrow?

What 3 things am I grateful for from my day?

1

2

3

HAYLEY BENNETT

7

The Balance Wheel

As you read at the beginning of this book, I had no balance in my life after the accident. I kept pushing myself, searching for a way back, a way to be like everyone else. What I wasn't doing was accepting who 'I' was and what 'I' needed to get through my day. I still re-check in; I use the wheel regularly particularly when life feels overwhelming. I check to see if work has taken over, if I'm not doing enough exercise or not had enough fun time with friends and family.

The key to managing anxiety and stress is to have a balanced life, this doesn't mean a perfect life, it doesn't mean everything has to go to plan or you need to be good and perfect all the time. It means having the things around you that help you get through life, it means learning to understand what you need for that day, week or month.

When we work with this resilience model *'My Balance Wheel'* meaning your wheel, your life, we can build a resilience to the circumstances around us, the things we can't control. As

I said earlier in the book, resilience is the capacity to recover from difficulties.

Research by Emmy E. Warner and Ruth S. Smith in 1989, shows that people with these qualities were more resilient:

- Problem solving ability
- Emotional support from outside the immediate family
- The belief that one can impact one's own destiny
- The ability to get on with others

A resilient person:

> *Loves well by having a loving and caring relationship in their life, works well by being successful in their job, plays well by having hobbies and enjoys leisure time and expects a positive future for their life*

Day 4 – Toolkit

Start your day with 5 things you are grateful for:

1

2

3

4

5

What is missing in your life?

MY BALANCE WHEEL

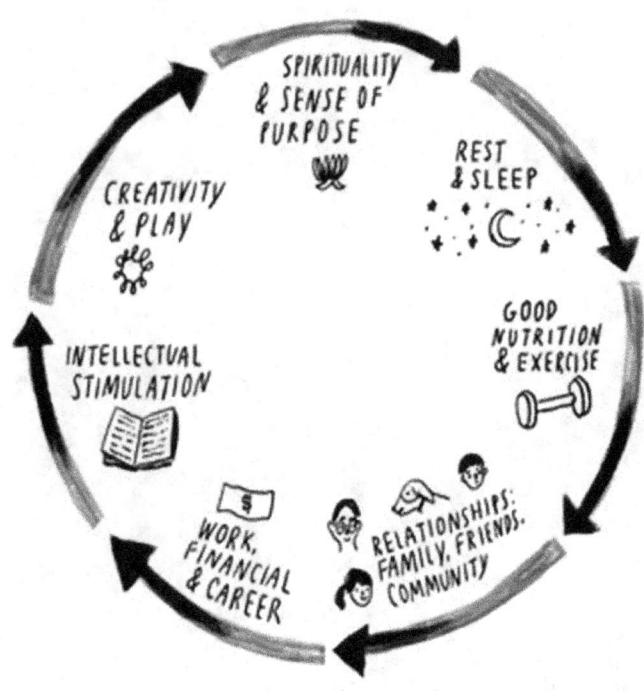

Take a look at the balance wheel and see what is missing in your life

Rest and Sleep
Sleep
Did you know that when we haven't had enough sleep it is like we are drunk? We are not reacting to a situation with a clear head, so a good night's sleep always helps. When we are tired the brain struggles to function and we will find it hard to cope with any decisions.

Rest/Relaxation
Learning relaxation techniques can help you with the mental and physical feelings of fear. It can help just to drop your shoulders and breathe deeply. Or imagine yourself in a relaxing place. You could also try learning things like yoga, Tai Chi or meditation. Taking timeout to read a book, stop and just listen to some music.

Complementary therapies
Some people find that complementary therapies or exercises, such as relaxation techniques, meditation, yoga, Tai Chi, reflexology, massage, acupuncture, etc. can help relax and deal with anxiety.

Good nutrition and exercise
Exercise
Increase the amount of exercise you do. Exercise requires some concentration, and this can take your mind off your fear and anxiety. Do at least 30 mins a day of some sort of exercise, this doesn't have to be all high intensity exercising, it can be walking, stretching, gardening.

Healthy eating

Eat lots of fruit and vegetables, try to avoid too much sugar. As sugar creates fluctuations in your blood sugar which can give you anxious feelings. Try to avoid drinking too much tea and coffee, as caffeine can increase anxiety levels.

Avoid alcohol, or drink in moderation

It's very common for people to drink when they feel nervous. Some people call alcohol 'Dutch courage', but the aftereffects of alcohol can make you feel even more afraid or anxious. We also use it to help us relax, but it can become a crutch.

Community, friends, family and relationships

These are a key aspect to a balanced happy life, no one person can be there all the time but each one has a unique role to play. Call on them when you need support and help, don't shut yourself away. Problems always feel bigger when they are alone in our heads and not shared. As they say, 'A problem shared is a problem halved.'

Work, financial and career

Having work give us purpose, I'm not just talking about paid work, be a mother, a carer or volunteering are just as important. Make sure your finances are in order; not dealing with bills that need paying, over spending, juggling money can cause us anxiety and stress.

Intellectual stimulation

Using our brain helps stimulate not just the mind but the body as well. Avoid sitting in front of the TV watching endless programmes, try and change things up, do some reading, listening to podcast, talks - Ted talks and videos. Try learning something new, sign up for a course, workshop either online, at night school, or at weekend.

Creativity and play

Be creative, do the things you love, write, draw, make something or do some photography. Have fun, laugh and go out and play. The happier we are with ourselves, the happier we are with life. If we have our own life in balance and feel happy in ourselves, we have less need to control every situation and then the fear and anxiety will start to fade away.

Faith, spirituality and sense of purpose

If you are religious or spiritual, this can give you a way of feeling connected to something bigger than yourself. Faith can provide a way of coping with everyday stress, and attending church and other faith groups can connect you with a valuable support network. When we have faith or a belief in something bigger than us, we have a sense of purpose and when we have a sense of purpose, we have motivation, drive and a goal.

Meditation 3 - Your Meadow

This meditation can be used at any time to help you relax, feel calm and clear your mind.

- Sit quietly and comfortably and close your eyes.
- Take a few deep breaths
- In front of you, there is a big pot and into this pot you need to put everything you no longer need or want, all your fears, worries and negativities.
- When you have finished, I would like you to put a lid onto your pot and ask for it to be taken away, changed into positivity and used for good whenever it is needed.
- Now imagine a golden bubble coming around yourself – Gold is the highest form of protection so this bubble will protect you, it will only allow good to come in.
- Fill your bubble with a positive colour. Breathe in the colour until it fills your whole body, from the top of your head to the tips of your toes – No Black, Red or Grey.
- In front of you is a light pathway, this path will lead you up to your meadow, follow the path.
- This is your meadow; it is a safe place. No one may enter your meadow unless you invite them.
- As you step into your meadow, you will hear the birds sing, see the butterflies dancing and feel the sun shining.
- As you walk through your meadow, look around, take it all in. Enjoy the peace and calmness.

- In your meadow there is a bench, walk over to your bench and take a seat.
- This is a nice place you can come to and just sit and have some peace.
- Stay here a while.....

- Now start walking back through your meadow to your path.
- Walk up your path and back into the room.

About my Day

Complete the questions below at the **END** of your day.

Today was a good/bad day for me because....

What did I learn from my day?

What can I change for tomorrow?

What 3 things am I grateful for from my day?

1

2

3

8

Reflection, Realisation and Relaxation

Reflection

What is reflection?

"...the way that we learn from an experience in order to understand and develop practice" (Jasper 2003)

We can reflect on everyday problems and situations:

- What went well?
- What didn't? and Why?
- How do I feel about it?

Reflection is a means of processing thoughts and feelings about an incident, or a difficult day...and gives us a chance to come to terms with our thoughts and feelings about it. Reflection can be particularly useful in dealing with a difficult or challenging situation.

This type of reflection may take place when we have had time to stand back from something, or talk it through, as in: 'on reflection, I think you might be right', or 'on second thoughts, I realise I was upset because...'

Realisation

This type of more focused reflection will lead to realisation. When we have the realisation, we can then find a new way of reacting or approaching the situation.

We have started doing this on a daily basis through the book in the *About My Day* section. So, doing a weekly journal in this chapter should come easier to you.

Day 5 – Toolkit

Start your day with 5 things you are grateful for:

1

2

3

4

5

Weekly Journal

What is reflective writing?

Reflective writing is evidence of reflective thinking.
Reflective thinking and writing can be organised into two stages:

- Looking closely at what happened, including your thoughts, feelings and reactions at the time; analysing what happened in depth, or from different perspectives.
- Thinking carefully about what you have learned from the whole reflective process and how your understanding has developed, and finally, identifying key points to take forward for future development, both personal and professional.

Writing a weekly journal can help with this. Look back on your week and reflect. Look at your *About my Day* sections from the last few days and write down how you have got on, what realisations you have had and what tools and techniques worked for you.

Relaxation

Reflexology

Reflexology has been a big part of my life and it started my career as a therapist. My son has grown up with it being part of his life too. I remember my first week at college and coming home in the evening with pen marks on my feet. We'd been drawing on each other's feet learning the different reflexology points. I was so proud of myself that I was learning something new after the accident and I wanted to show my son. He was about 5 years old at the time, I laid him down on the sofa, put his feet up, I had my towels laid out, my talcum powder ready (we use cream now a days) and I started. He giggled and moved around, as all children do but then he stopped and said to me.

"I want re-ology mum"

"This is reflexology" I replied

"NO, I want you to draw on my feet!"

What more could I say! I stopped what I was doing and drew on his feet, I was still learning, I was repeating what I had done at college all day. Over the last 20 years my son has used reflexology to help himself through life.

So, what is reflexology?

Reflexology is a natural healing system which uses the pressure points in the feet to correct imbalances in the body. By treating the whole body, we can clear the pathways to the mind, body and spirit. This will help relax and re-balance the body, boost your energy and restore the immune system.

OK; let's make it more basic:

By working on the pressure points in the feet or hands this will send blood, oxygen and energy up the body to the needed areas. This helps restore and balance the body. Reflexology is a treatment mainly done on the feet, but it can also be done on the hands, ears and face.

Reflexology helps with many different elements such as Back pain, Arthritis, Asthma, Stress, Infertility, Pregnancy, Fatigue, Insomnia, IBS, Headaches, Cancer, Thyroid and other hormonal problems. But here in the book I'm going to show you some self-help hand reflexology.

Self-help on your hands

Work one hand at a time, using the other hand to work the reflexes, then swap hands.

Make sure you work both hands, put a little bit of cream on your hands so you don't get skin on skin burns. try this for 5 mins a day

HAYLEY BENNETT

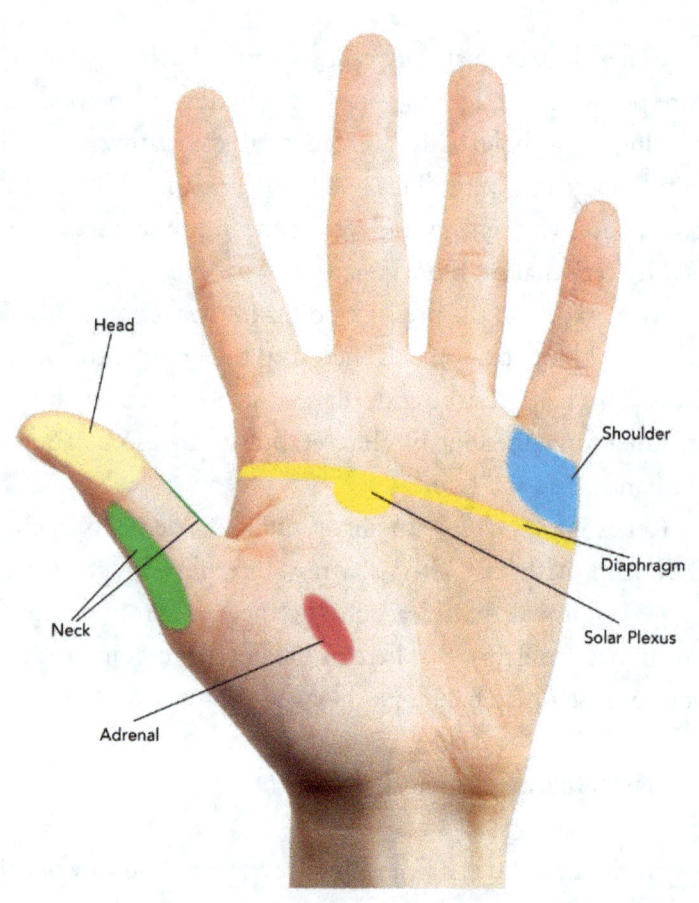

Diaphragm and Solar Plexus - Yellow - Relaxation and stress

1. Use your thumb to push across the yellow line (Diaphragm) on the opposite hand. Do this 2 or 3 times.
2. Then go to the centre yellow dot (Solar Plexus) and make slow circular movements.
3. Press gently into the solar plexus point and take 3 deep breaths, in through your nose and out through your mouth.

Head, Neck and shoulders - Cream, Green, and Blue - Releasing tension

1. Use your thumb to massage over the cream area (Head)
2. Use your thumb to push firmly along both green areas (Neck)
3. Use your thumb to massage firmly over the blue area (Shoulders)

Adrenal – Pink – Boost Energy or calm your energy down

1. Use the thumb to gently press and rotate over the pink dot (Adrenals) in the soft area between the thumb and first finger. (This point can feel tender).

HAYLEY BENNETT

9

The tools for your toolkit

Here are all the tools you have learnt in this book so far. You can use them in your everyday life. I'm not saying you have to use all of them on one day. Trying to do them all on top of your normal day will cause you more anxiety so just pick one or two. Choose the ones you feel work for you and you need on that day, use your gut feeling, go with what feels right. You can always add more in later when these become a habit or you can swap to a different one when something new comes up you have to deal with.

In most houses there is a toolkit, it is full of different tools. The things we use regularly are on the top section, e.g. screwdrivers and Allen keys. Then underneath we have the things we don't use all the time, e.g. a saw, drill and hammer but we still have them in the kit for when they are needed.

The *Toolkit for Anxiety and Stress - The Toolkit for Living*, works the same, we take out what we need, when we need it.

Remember; we have to hear something up to 8 times or more for us to learn it and it takes 21 days to form a new habit.

So, if you have a bad day or 'fall off the wagon' so to speak, just pick yourself up and start afresh the next day.

> *Each day is a new beginning!*

Start your day with a positive action:
5 Things to be grateful for

Focus on:
What sort of day you want to have?
What are the things or people you need to achieve it?

Check in at the end of your day:
How did my day go?
What did I learn from it good or bad?

Look at what drains you
Go back to the list, breakdown all the things you do and see what is draining you, see how you can change it.

Balance Wheel
Review your Balance Wheel to see what is missing/lacking, maybe you need to bring in a little more of one of the sections to help you feel more balanced.

Write a daily or weekly Journal
Look back on your day or week and reflect, write down how you have got on, what realisations you have had, what tools and techniques worked for you.

Hand Reflexology
Work on your hands when you are feeling anxious or you are having a panic attack or just need to unwind and relax.

Sit and Breathe
You can do either one or both of these breathing exercises to help you calm down, release your tension and fears or re-balance the brain.

Take a few deep and loud breaths
Alternate nostril breathing

Meditations
1 - The Bubble
2 - Your Meadow

HAYLEY BENNETT

Congratulations! You have completed Part One of this book, you now have all the tools you need to have a calm and productive day.

If you feel you need some more time to work on these tools, keep practising until you feel comfortable and happy them.

Ready for the next step?

In Part Two of this book there is a complete breakdown and plan of how you can achieve the next step in life, your goals and dreams.

Working towards the life you want

Part Two

Introduction

Now you have control of your anxiety and stress and it isn't running your life, you get to choose what next. You get to do all the things you dreamed of: changing your job, moving house, losing weight, getting fit, running a marathon, writing that book your always wanted to do, taking a course or just getting your life in a healthy balance. Whatever it is, you can't achieve it if you don't have a clear vision and plan. It's easy to start something and then drop it after a few weeks or months when life gets in the way or we hit a mental wall and we just stop doing it.

But if we break down the goal or dream, it helps us work through all these challenges and having awareness of our blocks and our strong points we can work with them, instead of against them and we can achieve the end result we desire.

Balance is the key to everything.
What we do, think, say, eat, feel, they all
require awareness
and through this awareness we can grow.
~Kio Fresco

In each of the following section there will be a number of questions that you will need to answer. Writing them down is a big part of getting a clear picture of what you want and staying focused. These questions are here to start you thinking, to help you to understand where you are now and where you are heading.

There are no right or wrong answers and it doesn't matter if you don't answer some of the questions but try your best. Be open and honest with yourself as this will help you get the most out of your workshop.

Plus, there will be a bonus sections to help you stay really focused on your goals and dreams.

10

Know your vision

Visioning is familiar to many of us, but how many actually take the time to do it?

- Do you have a 10-year plan?
- A 5-year plan?
- How about a one-year plan?
- If you have one personally, do you have one for your business?
- If for your business, how about personally?
- Do they align?
- Do your values translate across both plans?

Clarifying your vision is one of the most powerful ways to bring immediate change to your life. But many people struggle to discover their vision. Follow this simple plan and you will be on your way to creating and living a vision focused on the things most important to you.

When you live by your vision, everything changes. But without a vision, you'll be stuck in boredom, hope will dwindle, work will be monotonous, and relationships will be shallow.

Creating a Vision

The reason so few of us live out our vision is because we don't know where to start. Vision begins with dreaming. Not 'pie in the sky' dreaming like, "I want 10 Ferrari's and 8 vacation houses." As we learnt earlier in the book '*Things*' don't make us happy and they do nothing to motivate us to live our lives.

Visions are about hopes, dreams, and aspirations.

I'm talking about visions like:

- I want to lose the weight, so I can have more energy to play with my children or grandkids.
- I want to eat healthy and exercise more, so I can show and teach my children how to live and have a healthy life.
- I want to get the promotion at work, so I have more money and I can live comfortably without the stresses of my finances.
- I want to leave my job and work for myself, so I have more time for myself and the family.
- I want to change my job and do something that helps people more.

A real dream is about living for something *that's bigger than yourself*. It's your life's purpose, your mission, the reason you were created. What kind of legacy will you leave? What impact do you want to make in the lives of others around you? How can you change the world?

I believe that discovering, and living your vision is a *Spiritual Experience*. There is something very special hidden inside your vision and when you discover this treasure, it changes you forever. That treasure is the reason you were created and put on this earth.

> *Vision is the art of seeing things invisible.–*
> *Jonathan Swift*

All Your Life You've Been Fighting Yourself

Here's a scary reality: when you are not clear on your vision you are living *against yourself*. You're living in opposition to who you really are and what you're supposed to be doing with your one and only amazing life!

The truth is that you are here for a reason. You are created with intention and unique gifts to share with the people around you. Discovering who you are and what you're supposed to be doing is the most important thing you will ever do.

Now, don't get overwhelmed. If you don't discover your complete life purpose through this process, don't sweat it. We live out our vision in phases and if you are only able to see a small part of your vision now, that's perfectly fine. Live that piece with all your heart and more vision will come with time. What's most important is to go through this process of discovery and start living for whatever vision you grab a hold of. The rest will come.

The 2 most common obstacles I see people trip over as they try to come up with their vision are:

1. They give up because they can't see the entire picture of their vision.
2. FEAR and FAILURE. They are afraid that once they commit themselves and write down the vision they might fail.

Let me encourage you to push though these issues. *The only failure is not trying.* Once you start living your vision and see it become reality, a whole new world opens to you and you will never be the same.

A vision pulls people forward. It projects a clear image of a possible future. It generates the enthusiasm and energy to strive toward the goal. To achieve something, we need to know what it is we really want and how it will make us feel went we have it. These are key steps to staying focused when things get a little tricky and we want to give up.

Complete the questions below to know your vision

What is my Goal or Dream?

What will I achieve from this Goal or Dream?

What can I see myself doing/having/being after I have achieved my Goal or Dream?

How will my mind, body and life feel after achieving my Goal or Dream?

Is my Goal or Dream realistic?

If not, how can I change it and make it realistic?

Bonus exercise:

Start making a vision board, poster or box
This will help you stay focused on your Goal or Dream.

What is a Vision Board/Poster or Box?

A vision board, poster or box is a visualisation tool which refers to a board of any sort, a poster you have created or a box full of your vision used to build a collage of words and pictures that represent your goals and dreams.

By placing visual representations of your goals into one space, you can easily visualise them frequently. Remembering to look at them daily and imagine them as if they have already come true is one of the best ways to activate the Law of Attraction - The law of attraction is the ability to attract into our lives whatever we are focusing on. The mind is like a magnet, what we focus on, we attract. It is believed that regardless of age, nationality, or religious belief, we are all susceptible to the laws which govern the Universe, including the Law of Attraction. It is the Law of Attraction that uses the power of the mind to translate whatever is in our thoughts and materialise them into reality. So, if we picture what we want and focus on it, we can create it in our life. We can start to see ourselves doing and having it. We can start to live and breathe it and make it real.

Start collecting pictures, words, quotes from the internet, magazines, etc that represent your Goal or Dream, also find a board or box. You can create your vision board, poster on your computer and print it out if you prefer but just start collecting today.

11

Know the consequences of not achieving your vision

What does the word consequences mean?

Consequences: Results of a particular action or situation, often ones that are bad or not convenient.

It is so easy to give up on our goals and dreams because we've not stopped and taken the time to look at the consequences of not achieving them. When we do take the time, we bring it to the forefront of our mind, we remind ourselves of the reasons we are doing it. It is so easy to forget all these things when it becomes too hard or inconvenient and we just want to give up.

In this section we look at what happens if you don't make these changes, how it will make you feel and who it affects.

Complete the questions below to understand the consequences of not achieving your vision

What happens if I DON'T make these changes?

What will I feel like and how will I look?

What will I be unable to do and who else will be affected by this?

What will be the impact on those I care about?

Bonus exercise:

Start putting your vision board, poster or box together. (If you are doing a vision box, you can stick things to the outside of your box as well as putting some inside)

You can add more things to your vision board/poster or box at any time to help you stay focused.

How Do You Use a Vision Board for Goal-Setting?

The best way to achieve your goals is to keep them at the forefront of your mind, so you're always looking for ways to move closer to them – and a vision board is the perfect tool to help you do that.

By putting a vision board somewhere you can see it every day, you will prompt yourself to visualise your ideal life on a regular basis. That's important because visualisation activates the creative powers of your subconscious mind and programs your brain to notice available resources that were always there but escaped your notice.

Through the Law of Attraction, visualisation also magnetizes and attracts to you the people, resources, and opportunities you need to achieve your goal.

By adding a visualisation practice to your daily routine, you will naturally become more motivated to reach your goals. You'll start to notice you are unexpectedly doing things that move you closer to your ideal life. Suddenly, you find yourself volunteering to take on more responsibility at work, speaking out at staff meetings, asking more directly for what you want, and taking more risks in your personal and professional life – and experiencing bigger pay-offs.

12

Know your reason for your vision!

What Is your "Reason" or your "Why"?

In today's world we hear a lot about knowing our 'Why', know why you are doing your business, know why you are achieving that goal. But your why is the same as your reason.

Your *'Reason'* is a statement of purpose that describes the reason you're doing what you do!

When we know our reason for our goals or dreams, we have purpose. When we have purpose, we have something to drive us and when we have something to drive us, we have more chance of achieving it.

In this section we look at what happens if you do make these changes, how you will feel and look, what you are able to do and who benefits. We also take a look at how your future will look when you achieve your goal or dream.

Complete the questions below to know your reason for your vision.

What will happen if I DO make these changes?

What will I feel and look like?

How will I feel about myself?

What will I be able to do and who else will benefit from it?

What will be the impact on those I care about?

What will my life look like in a year?

What will my life look like in 5 years?

Bonus exercise:

Meditation - Feel and See your Vision

EMOTIONS and FEELINGS help to strengthen neural pathways - the habit-forming parts of the brain.

- Close your eyes - visualise your goal or dream, how good does it feel?
- Sit in the feeling, hold it, remember how good it feels!!
- Smile!!! From the inside out.
- Allow your body and your mind to glow.

13

Know and understand the things that are holding you back.

We all hit a point when we want to give up on something and we start hearing negative chatter in our heads or we start to make excuses and find ways not to carry on. By knowing and understanding the things that hold us back, we can work with them and keep moving forward towards our goal.

One of the biggest reasons we hold ourselves back are our limiting beliefs about ourselves. Example: 'I'm not good enough'. 'Everyone knows I'm a fake.' .'I never finish anything, so why bother'. 'I don't deserve or need all the money, so why bother going for the promotion'. 'I don't deserve to be happy' and so many more. We might not realise it is coming from these beliefs as we mask them with default habits.

- Going to the fridge or cupboard for another snack, when you're on a diet.
- Sitting watching TV when you have things to do.

- Having another drink to mask the loneliness, the inner pain, the sadness, etc
- Making life busy and stressful
- Making excuses
- Blaming others

In this section we will look at the ways you cope with challenges and stress and go into more detail about negative – automatic – thoughts and how you can change them.

Complete the questions below to know and understand the things that are holding you back.

What ways do I cope with emotional challenges or with being stressed?

Is this reaction a positive or negative one?

Will this reaction stop me achieving my Goal or Dream?

> *Beware of what your mind is doing.
> Suffering comes from the mind and how we
> see the situation.*

Stress - Anxiety - Worry

Stress is wanting the present moment to be something it's not.

Anxiety and worry are creating a narrative in the mind of what *might* happen and then staying focused on it. By staying focused on the story in our head, our emotions kick in. Example: fear, this reinforces the narrative.

Negative – Automatic - Thoughts or NATs

NATs are thoughts that seem to just pop into your head without warning, they often trigger negative feelings and drive your behaviour in unhelpful directions.

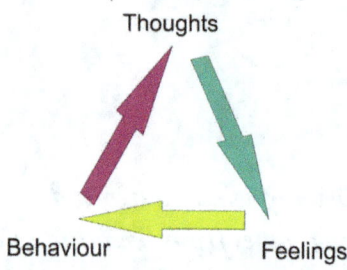

List all your negative thoughts and feelings.........

Developing balanced thinking can break this pattern of negative thinking and feelings. Here are some questions you can ask yourself when you feel you are slipping into negative thoughts and feelings.

- **What evidence is there that this thought is true?**
- **What evidence is there that this thought is not true?**
- **What would I tell someone I loved if they were in this situation and had these thoughts?**
- **If my automatic thought is true, what is the worst that could happen?**
- **If my automatic thought is true, what is the best thing that could happen?**

Once evidence has been generated, combine it to form a more balanced thought. This thought will likely be much longer than the original NAT thought.

Bonus exercise:

Creating a new alternative thought to help break the negative behaviour.

Creating a new alternative thought, doesn't mean that we simply develop a new thought which is complete opposite of the negative; going from one extreme to the other is not particularly helpful or realistic. It is about creating a more balanced and realistic thought.

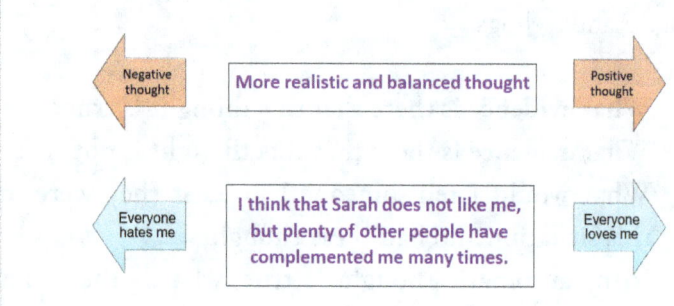

Once you have your negative thought, decide what the other extreme would be (going from the negative thought to a positive thought) and then, using the evidence for and against, try to create a balanced and realistic thought to work with.

You might want to ask the following questions:

- **Taking the information into account, is there an alternative way of thinking about the situation?**
- **Can someone I trust understand this situation in a different way?**

Pick a few of your negative thoughts or feelings and fill in the chart below.

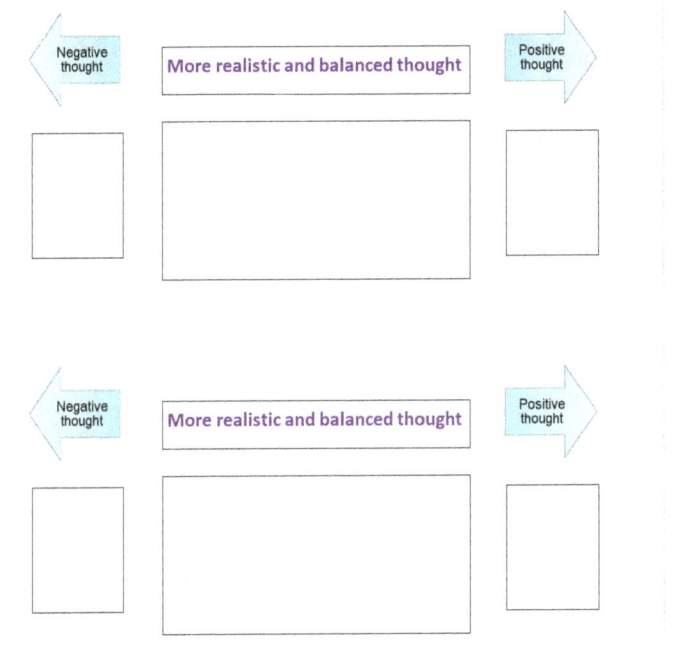

Another way of doing it is to put a possibility on the negative thought or belief to get a realistic one.

Instead of saying - *I can't do this!*

Say – *I can't do this, Yet!*

Or *I can't do 'X', but I can do 'Y'.*

HAYLEY BENNETT

14

Know your plan.

Vision summary brainstorm!

Complete the questions below to know your plan.

What exactly is it that I want to achieve?

Goal setting. It's in the detail:

Achieving your vision means setting goals. Without a practical plan it's hard to turn ideas into reality. Breaking down your goals into smaller achievable pieces prevents them from becoming overwhelming.

Remember to ask yourself these kinds of questions:

What needs to happen in order for me to achieve my vision?

What specific goals will I need to set?

What different steps will I have to take to get there?

Your Strategy:

Are my goals realistic in terms of my commitment and time?

What resources do I need? (Finances, equipment, time, childcare, etc.) How will I get them?

What will I be unable to do and who else will be affected by this?

Who do I need on-board to achieve my goals?

What tools do I need to put in my tool box to help me to achieve my goals?

As you do this, consider previous patterns. What has worked well and what hasn't?

When something didn't work well, what were the triggers?

What can you implement to prevent that happening again?

Action

Any achievement, no matter how great, when you break it down it is just a series of steps. Putting one foot in front of the other to accomplish each of the goals, eventually takes you to your vision... your success....your happier you!!!

Sustainability and momentum

EMOTION helps to strengthen neural pathways - the habit-forming parts of the brain. So, celebrate small victories - throw yourself an internal party when you complete any of your actions or goals.

- Close your eyes - feel the feeling you feel, how good does it feel after achieving your action or goal?
- Sit in the feeling, hold it, remember how good it feels!!
- Smile!!! From the inside out. Allow your body and your mind to glow.

Measure your progress - Take the time to look back at what you have written and see how far you have come. Every single step is a step in the right direction.

Try and do your visualisation every day. Keeping your ambition at the forefront of your mind will help make that far-away goal more of a reality.

Make notes of what's working and what's not. Analyse successes and failures to help you plan the next step.

Don't be afraid to revisit and refine goals and strategies as you learn more about yourself and love yourself more.

SELF-HELP TOOLKIT FOR ANXIETY AND STRESS

Formula for success for any part of your life.

SUMMARY

VISION

- What do I really want?
- How will this be useful for me?

GOAL

- What are all the things that need to happen in order for me to achieve this.

STRATEGY

- What are all the component parts of my goals?
- What is the best order to tackle them?
- What resources do I need?
- What has worked well or not well in the past?

ACTION

- What small steps can I take each day to get me closer to my goals and vision?
- What am I going to do and when?

HAYLEY BENNETT

Congratulations!
You have completed part two this book and you now have all the tools to move forward with your goals and dreams.

Notes:

Notes:

Notes:

Bibliography

Courtney E. Ackerman, MA. 31-10-2020 - What Is Happiness and Why Is It Important? Positive Psychology available at https://positivepsychology.com/what-is-happiness/ retrieved 2021

Courtney E. Ackerman, MA. 05-02-2021 - What is Gratitude and Why Is It So Important? Positive Psychology available at https://positivepsychology.com/gratitude-appreciation/ retrieved 2021

Kempton, Beth. Wasbi Sabi, Japanese wisdom for a perfectly imperfect life. Great Britain: Piatkus 2018

Brown, Brené. 202, LinkedIn https://www.linkedin.com/in/brenebrown/detail/recent-activity/

Cheryl Richardson. Take Time for Your Life, A Personal Coach's 7-Step Program for Creating the Life You Want. Broadway Books Jan 16 2000

Sadhguru, Sep 26, 2016. What is Happiness? YouTube: https://www.youtube.com/watch?v=VAn8t80lclM

Tim Ferriss. Feb 10, 2020. Tim Ferriss and Brené Brown on Self-Acceptance and Complacency. YouTube. https://www.youtube.com/watch?v=znRLbEcFrRU

Holden, Robert. PhD. Be Happy, Release the power of happiness in YOU. United Kingdom. Hay House UK Ltd 2009

DEFINITIONS found at Dictioary.com, www.dictionary.com. Urban Dictionary, www.urbandictionary.com. Oxford English Dictionary, www.oed.com

Acknowledgments

I am so grateful to all the people that have been there for me through my life, the ones that have supported me through the good and bad times. But this book wouldn't be here if it wasn't for all the support and help from Kered, John and Samuel.

Kered for all the time she spent helping me get this book to where it is, for believing in me and her unconditional friendship.

John for being there for me, listening to me and encouraging me.

Samuel for supporting and helping me navigate through the world of self-publishing.

Thank you to everyone who read through my book and proof read it for me.

I can't thank you enough, all my love. x

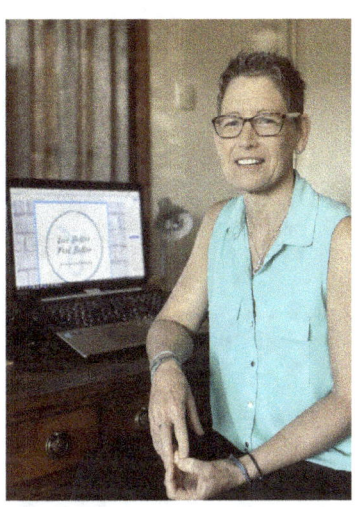

I am the owner of Hayley Bennett Wellbeing – Reflexologist, Shift – Creation coach, Speaker and Author. I have been working with clients since 2002 and I have been practicing what I teach personally since 1993.

I provide individuals and companies with tools, techniques and support to help manage their wellness and mental health and help create a life and career you don't want to escape from.

I live in the beautiful Cotswolds but have also lived in Bermuda and Cyprus and my passion for travelling and seeing the world, meeting new and interesting people has been a big driving force to create an online business and provide courses, one-to-one treatments, mentoring and talks around the world.

This book is the culmination of 28 years of studying, personal tools and teaching. I hope it helps you as much as it has helped me. To get in touch and be a part of my motivational and mindset emails you can email me on hello@hayleybennettwellbeing.com

WHAT IS LIVE BETTER – FEEL BETTER – WORK BETTER?

I am the founder of the Live Better – Feel Better – Work Better Group where I provide a safe place for people to be honest and open about the things they are struggling with. This isn't a place to moan and complain, it's a place to find tools and techniques to get through life's ups and downs. In this group I provide monthly support and mentoring. Master classes, Meditations, Guest Speakers and Live Chats.

I believe if we Live Better, we will Feel Better mentally and physically and then we Work Better, either in our job/career or as parents.

To be part of the group and have constant support around you go to: https://hayleybennettwellbeing.com/

WHAT IS SHIFT – CREATION COACHING?

Shift - Creation Coaching is designed to help you understand the mind, body and spirit, and to see the things that are holding you back. You will learn new tools for your 'Tool box of Life' and it will help you create a balanced and happier life.

The one year or 6-months package will support you through your journey. You will receive a one-to-one, online sessions with me, Hayley Bennett every week for the first month, then every two weeks for the second month, then once a month for the rest of the year or 6-months. I will be here to help guide you through anything you are struggling with, we will set goals and action plans so you learn how to put everything you learn into practice. At the end of the year or 6-months you will have shifted your mindset and created a life you deserve. Plus, you will leave with a plan to help you carry on and move forward after the program is finished.

By helping you discover the things that are holding you back and help you to redesign your inner thinking space and

WHAT IS SHIFT – CREATION COACHING?

shifting your mindset. You can be the person you are meant to be and create a life and career you don't want to escape from.

For a free consultation and to see if Shift – Creation Coaching is right for you. Email me on: hello@hayleybennettwellbeing.com

WHAT IS REFLEXOLOGY?

Reflexology is a non-invasive complementary health therapy that can be effective in promoting deep relaxation and wellbeing; by reducing stress in people's lives can be key in optimising good health and building resilience. It is a touch therapy that is based on the theory that different points on the feet, lower leg, hands, face or ears correspond with different areas of the body and reflexologists work these points and areas.

However reflexology is viewed, there can be no doubt that what it does provide is a period of time for relaxation where the client has one to one attention and supportive touch in an empathetic listening environment. Reflexology can be used safely alongside standard healthcare to promote better health for their clients.

What's the main theory behind reflexology?

The theory of reflexology is that all the systems and organs of the whole body are mirrored or reflected in smaller peripheral areas, for example the feet, hands, ears and face.

The reflexologist simply works those reflected areas with their sensitive fingers, aiming to bring those areas back to balance and therefore aiding the body to work as well as it can. Reflexology very much works on an individual basis; the reflexologist provides professional facilitation of your body's own potential for well-being.

A brief history of Western reflexology

Whilst the art of reflexology dates back to Ancient Egypt, India and China, this therapy was not introduced to the West until Dr William Fitzgerald developed 'Zone therapy' in the early 1900s. He believed that reflex areas on the feet and hands were linked to other areas and organs of the body within the same zone.

In the 1930's, Eunice Ingham further developed this zone therapy into what is known as reflexology. Her opinion was that congestion or tension in any part of the foot is mirrored in the corresponding part of the body.

Physical and emotional benefits of Reflexology

- **Helps release aches, pain e.g. Back, neck, shoulder and arthritis**
- **Promotes relaxation which relieves stress, fear, anger and anxiety**
- Can boost the immune system
- Can help reduce fluid retention and swelling
- Helps manage hormone imbalances e.g. Menopause, PMS, Infertility, Thyroid

- Can boost energy levels
- Assist sleep
- Helps through pregnancy
- Helps to release headaches and IBS
- Helps with Asthma
- A good support through cancer treatment
- Eliminates Allergies
- Help to keep a positive outlook and a sense of well-being
- Releases emotion Blockages

To find a fully qualified reflexologist near you go to the Association of Reflexologist website: https://www.aor.org.uk/custom/far-search/

www.ingramcontent.com/pod-product-compliance
Lightning Source LLC
Chambersburg PA
CBHW070909080526
44589CB00013B/1230